QUICK REFERENCE GUIDE FOR CLINICIANS
2008 UPDATE

Treating Tobacco Use And Dependence

U.S. Department of
Health and Human Services
Public Health Service

To All Clinicians

The Public Health Service-sponsored Clinical Practice Guideline *Treating Tobacco Use and Dependence: 2008 Update,* on which this Quick Reference Guide for Clinicians is based, was developed by a multidisciplinary, non-Federal panel of experts in collaboration with a consortium of tobacco cessation representatives, consultants, and staff. Panel members, Federal liaisons, and guideline staff were as follows:

Guideline Panel

Michael C. Fiore, MD, MPH
(Panel Chair)
Carlos Roberto Jaén, MD, PhD, FAAFP
(Panel Vice Chair)
Timothy B. Baker, PhD
(Senior Scientist)
William C. Bailey, MD
Neal Benowitz, MD
Susan J. Curry, PhD
Sally Faith Dorfman, MD
Erika S. Froelicher, PhD, RN, MA, MPH
Micahael G. Goldstein, MD
Cheryl G. Healton, DrPH
Patricia Nez Henderson, MD, MPH

Richard B. Heyman, MD
Howard K. Koh, MD, MPH, FACP
Thomas E. Kottke, MD, MSPH
Harry A. Lando, PhD
Robert E. Mecklenburg, DDS, MPH
Robin J. Mermelstein, PhD
Patricia Dolan Mullen, DrPH
C. Tracy Orleans, PhD
Lawrence Robinson, MD, MPH
Maxine L. Stitzer, PhD
Anthony C. Tommasello, MS
Louise Villejo, MPH, CHES
Mary Ellen Wewers, PhD, RN

Guideline Liaisons

Ernestine W. Murray, RN, BSN, MAS (Project Officer), Agency for
    Healthcare Research and Quality
Glenn Bennett, MPH, CHES, National Heart, Lung, and Blood Institute
Stephen Heishman, PhD, National Institute on Drug Abuse
Corinne Husten, MD, MPH, Centers for Disease Control and Prevention
Glen Morgan, PhD, National Cancer Institute
Christine Williams, MEd, Agency for Healthcare Research and Quality

Guideline Staff

Bruce Christiansen, PhD (Project Director)
Megan E. Piper, PhD (Project Scientist)
Victor Hasselblad, PhD (Project Statistician)
David Fraser, MS (Project Coordinator)
Wendy Theobald, PhD (Editorial Associate)
Michael Connell, BS (Database Manager)
Cathlyn Leitzke, MSN, RN-C (Project Researcher)

An explicit science-based methodology was employed along with expert clinical judgment to develop recommendations on treating tobacco use and dependence. Extensive literature searches were conducted and critical reviews and syntheses were used to evaluate empirical evidence and significant outcomes. Peer review was undertaken to evaluate the validity, reliability, and utility of the guideline in clinical practice. See the complete Guideline (available at www.surgeongeneral.gov/tobacco/) for the methods, peer reviewers, references, and financial disclosure information.

This Quick Reference Guide for Clinicians presents summary points from the Clinical Practice Guideline. The guideline provides a description of the developmental process, through analysis and discussion of the available research, critical evaluation of the assumptions and knowledge of the field, and more complete information for health care decisionmaking. Decisions to adopt particular recommendations from either publication must be made by practitioners in light of available resources and circumstances presented by the individual patient.

As clinicians, you are in the frontline position to help your patients by asking two key questions: "Do you smoke?" and "Do you want to quit?," followed by use of the recommendations in this Quick Reference Guide for Clinicians.

QUICK REFERENCE GUIDE FOR CLINICIANS

Treating Tobacco Use and Dependence

U.S. Department of Health and Human Services
Public Health Service

April 2009

1

Abstract

The Quick Reference Guide for Clinicians contains strategies and recommendations from the Public Health Service-sponsored Clinical Practice Guideline *Treating Tobacco Use and Dependence: 2008 Update.* The guideline was designed to assist clinicians; smoking cessation specialists; and healthcare administrators, insurers, and purchasers in identifying and assessing tobacco users and in delivering effective tobacco dependence interventions. It was based on an exhaustive systematic review and analysis of the extant scientific literature from 1975–2007 and uses the results of more then 50 meta-analyses.

The Quick Reference Guide for Clinicians summarizes the guideline strategies for providing appropriate treatments for every patient. Effective treatments for tobacco dependence now exist, and every patient should receive at least minimal treatment every time he or she visits a clinician. The first step in the process—identification and assessment of tobacco use status—separates patients into three treatment categories: (1) tobacco users who are willing to quit should receive intervention to help in their quit attempt; (2) those who are unwilling to quit now should receive interventions to increase their motivation to quit; and (3) those who recently quit using tobacco should be provided relapse prevention treatment.

Suggested Citation

This document is in the public domain and may be used and reprinted without special permission. The Pubic Health Service appreciates citation as to source, and the suggested format is provided below:

Fiore MC, Jaén CR, Baker TB, et al. Treating Tobacco Use and Dependence: 2008 Update. Quick Reference Guide for Clinicians. Rockville, MD: U.S. Department of Health and Human Services. Public Health Service. April 2009.

Purpose

Tobacco is the single greatest cause of disease and premature death in America today, and is responsible for more than 435,000 deaths annually. About 20 percent of adult Americans currently smoke, and 4,000 children and adolescents smoke their first cigarette each day. The societal costs of tobacco-related death and disease approach $96 billion annually in medical expenses and $97 billion in lost productivity. However, more then 70 percent of all current smokers have expressed a desire to stop smoking; if they successfully quit, the result will be both immediate and long-term health improvements. Clinicians have a vital role to play in helping smokers quit.

The analyses contained within the Clinical Practice Guideline *Treating Tobacco Use and Dependence: 2008 Update* demonstrated that efficacious treatments for tobacco users exist and should become a part of standard care giving. Research also shows that delivering such treatments is cost-effective. In summary, the treatment of tobacco use and dependence presents the best and most cost-effective opportunity for clinicians to improve the lives of millions of Americans nationwide.

Key Findings

The guideline identified a number of key findings that clinicians should use:

1. Tobacco dependence is a chronic disease that often requires repeated intervention and multiple attempts to quit. Effective treatments exist, however, that can significantly increase rates of long-term abstinence.

2. It is essential that clinicians and healthcare delivery systems consistently identify and document tobacco use status and treat every tobacco user seen in a healthcare setting.

3. Tobacco dependence treatments are effective across a broad range of populations. Clinicians should encourage every patient willing to make a quit attempt to use the recommended counseling treatments and medications in the Guideline.

4. Brief tobacco dependence treatment is effective. Clinicians should offer every patient who uses tobacco at least the brief treatments shown to be effective in the Guideline.

3

5. Individual, group and telephone counseling are effective and their effectiveness increases with treatment intensity. Two components of counseling are especially effective and clinicians should use these when counseling patients making a quit attempt:

   ▸ Practical counseling (problem-solving/skills training)

   ▸ Social support delivered as part of treatment

6. There are numerous effective medications for tobacco dependence and clinicians should encourage their use by all patients attempting to quit smoking, except when medically contraindicated or with specific populations for which there is insufficient evidence of effectiveness (i.e., pregnant women, smokeless tobacco users, light smokers and adolescents).

   ▸ Seven first-line medications (5 nicotine and 2 non-nicotine) reliably increase long-term smoking abstinence rates:

   — Bupropion SR

   — Nicotine gum

   — Nicotine inhaler

   — Nicotine lozenge

   — Nicotine nasal spray

   — Nicotine patch

   — Varenicline

   ▸ Clinicians should also consider the use of certain combinations of medications identified as effective in the Guideline.

7. Counseling and medication are effective when used by themselves for treating tobacco dependence. However, the combination of counseling and medication is more effective than either alone. Thus, clinicians should encourage all individuals making a quit attempt to use both counseling and medication.

8. Telephone quitline counseling is effective with diverse populations and has broad reach. Therefore, clinicians and healthcare delivery systems should both ensure patient access to quitlines and promote quitline use.

9. If a tobacco user is currently unwilling to make a quit attempt, clinicians should use the motivational treatments shown in the Guideline to be effective in increasing future quit attempts.

10. Tobacco dependence treatments are both clinically effective and highly cost-effective relative to interventions for other clinical disorders. Providing coverage for these treatments increases quit rates. Insurers and purchasers should ensure that all insurance plans include the counseling and medication identified as effective in the Guideline as covered benefits.

Tobacco Dependence as a Chronic Health Condition

Tobacco dependence is a chronic health condition that often requires multiple, discrete interventions by a clinician or team of clinicians. The "5 A's" of treating tobacco dependence (Ask, Advise, Assess, Assist, and Arrange follow-up) is a useful way to understand tobacco dependence treatment and organize the clinical team to deliver that treatment. While a single clinician can provide all 5 A's, it is often more clinically and cost-effective to have the 5 A's implemented by a team of clinicians and ancillary staff. However when a team is used, coordination of efforts is essential with a single clinician retaining overall responsibility for the interventions. Clinician extenders such as quit lines, web-based interventions, local quit programs and tailored, self-help materials can often be, and should be, incorporated into the 5 A's approach. These treatment extenders can make clinical interventions more efficient.

This Quick Reference Guide for Clinicians is organized around the 5 A's. However, the clinical situation may suggest delivering these components in a different order or format. The following sections address the three main groups of tobacco users: (1) those who are willing to quit, (2) those who are unwilling to quit now, and (3) those who recently quit. This Quick Reference Guide is based on Guideline findings and includes many tables directly from the Guideline.

Table 1. The "5 A's" model for treating tobacco use and dependence

Ask about tobacco use	Identify and document tobacco use status of every patient at every visit.
Advise to quit	In a clear, strong and personalized manner urge every tobacco user to quit.
Assess	For current tobacco user, is the tobacco user willing to make a quit attempt at this time?
	For the ex-tobacco user, how recent did you quit and are there any challenges to remaining abstinent?
Assist	For the patient willing to make a quit attempt, offer medication and provide or refer for counseling or additional behavioral treatment to help the patient quit.
	For patients unwilling to quit at this time, provide motivational interventions designed to increase future quit attempts.
	For the recent quitter and any with remaining challenges, provide relapse prevention
Arrange	All those receiving the previous A's should receive followup.

Figure 1. The "5 A's": Treating Tobacco Dependence as a Chronic Disease

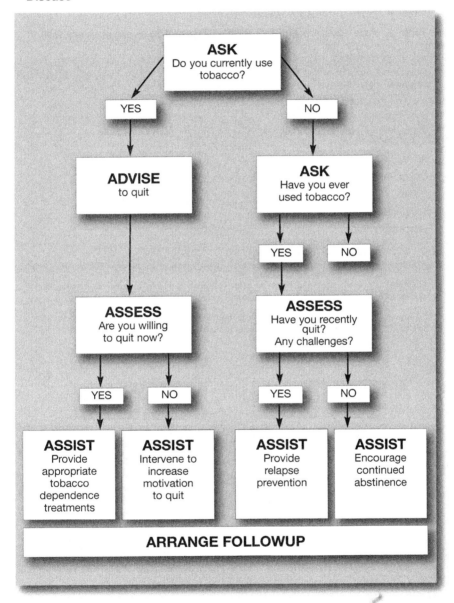

7

TOBACCO USERS WILLING TO QUIT

The "5 A's," Ask, Advise, Assess, Assist, and Arrange, are designed to be used with the smoker who is willing to quit.

Table 2. Ask—systematically identify all tobacco users at every visit

Action	Strategies for implementation
Implement an officewide system that ensures that, for EVERY patient at EVERY clinic visit, tobacco-use status is queried and documented.[a]	Expand the vital signs to include tobacco use or use an alternative universal identification system.[b]

VITAL SIGNS

Blood Pressure:_____

Pulse: _____ Weight: _____

Temperature: _____

Respiratory Rate: _____

Tobacco Use (circle one):   Current   Former   Never

[a] Repeated assessment is not necessary in the case of the adult who has never used tobacco or has not used tobacco for many years and for whom this information is clearly documented in the medical record.

[b] Alternatives to expanding the vital signs include using tobacco use status stickers on all patient charts or indicating tobacco use status via electronic medical records or computerized reminder systems.

Table 3. Advise—Strongly urge all tobacco users to quit

Action	Strategies for implementation
In a clear, strong, and personalized manner, urge every tobacco user to quit.	Advice should be: ■ Clear—"I think it is important for you to quit smoking (or using chewing tobacco) now, and I can help you." "Cutting down while you are ill is not enough." "Occasional or light smoking is still dangerous." ■ Strong—"As your clinician, I need you to know that quitting smoking is the most important thing you can do to protect your health now and in the future. The clinic staff and I will help you." ■ Personalized—Tie tobacco use to current symptoms and health concerns, and/or its social and economic costs, and/or the impact of tobacco use on children and others in the household. "Continuing to smoke makes your asthma worse, and quitting may dramatically improve your health. Quitting smoking may reduce the number of ear infections your child has."

Table 4. Assess—Determine willingness to make a quit attempt

Action	Strategies for implementation

Assess every tobacco user's willingness to make a quit attempt at the time.	Assess patient's willingness to quit: "Are you willing to give quitting a try?'
	■ If the patient is willing to make a quit attempt, provide assistance.
	  – If the patient will participate in an intensive treatment, deliver such a treatment or link/refer to an intensive intervention.
	  – If the patient is a member of a special population (e.g., adolescent, pregnant smoker, racial/ethnic minority), consider providing additional information.
	■ If the patient clearly states that he or she is unwilling to make a quit attempt at the time, provide an intervention shown to increase future quit attempts.

Table 5. Assist—Aid the patient in quitting (provide counseling and medication)

Action	Strategies for implementation
Help the patient with a quit plan.	A patient's preparations for quitting: ▪ **S**et a quit date. Ideally, the quit date should be within 2 weeks. ▪ **T**ell family, friends, and coworkers about quitting and request understanding and support. ▪ **A**nticipate challenges to the upcoming quit attempt, particularly during the critical first few weeks. These include nicotine withdrawal symptoms. ▪ **R**emove tobacco products from your environment. Prior to quitting, avoid smoking in places where you spend a lot of time (e.g., work, home, car). Make your home smoke-free.
Recommend the use of approved medication, except when contraindicated or with specific populations for which there is insufficient evidence of effectiveness (i.e., pregnant women, smokeless tobacco users, light smokers, and adolescents).	Explain how these medications increase quitting success and reduce withdrawal symptoms. FDA-approved medications include: bupropion SR, nicotine gum, nicotine inhaler, nicotine lozenge, nicotine nasal spray, nicotine patch, and varenicline. There is insufficient evidence to recommend medication for pregnant women, adolescents, smokeless tobacco users, and light smokers (< 10 cigarettes/day).
Provide practical counseling (problem-solving/skills training).	*Abstinence*. Striving for total abstinence is essential. Not even a single puff after the quit date. *Past quit experience*. Identify what helped and what hurt in previous quit attempts. Build on past success. *Anticipate triggers or challenges in the upcoming attempt*. Discuss challenges/triggers and how the patient will successfully overcome them (e.g., avoid triggers, alter routines).

10

Table 5. Assist—Aid the patient in quitting (provide counseling and medication) (continued)

Action	Strategies for implementation
	Alcohol. Because alcohol is associated with relapse, the patient should consider limiting/abstaining from alcohol while quitting. (Note that reducing alcohol intake could precipitate withdrawal in alcohol-dependent persons.)
	Other smokers in the household. Quitting is more difficult when there is another smoker in the household. Patients should encourage housemates to quit with them or to not smoke in their presence.
Provide intratreatment social support.	Provide a supportive clinical environment while encouraging the patient in his or her quit attempt. "My office staff and I are available to assist you." "I'm recommending treatment that can provide ongoing support."
Provide supplementary materials, including information on quitlines.	*Sources:* Federal agencies, nonprofit agencies, national quitline network (1-800-QUIT-NOW), or local/state/tribal health departments/quitlines.
	Type: Culturally/racially/educationally/age-appropriate for the patient.
	Location: Readily available at every clinician's workstation.

ASSIST COMPONENT—PROVIDING COUNSELING

Counseling should include teaching practical problem solving skills and providing support and encouragement.

Table 6. Common elements of practical counseling

Practical counseling (problem-solving/skills training) treatment component	Examples
Recognize danger situations – Identify events, internal states, or activities that increase the risk of smoking or relapse.	■ Negative affect and stress. ■ Being around other tobacco users. ■ Drinking alcohol. ■ Experiencing urges. ■ Smoking cues and availability of cigarettes.
Develop coping skills – Identify and practice coping or problem-solving skills. Typically, these skills are intended to cope with danger situations.	■ Learning to anticipate and avoid temptation and trigger situations. ■ Learning cognitive strategies that will reduce negative moods. ■ Accomplishing lifestyle changes that reduce stress, improve quality of life, and reduce exposure to smoking cues. ■ Learning cognitive and behavioral activities to cope with smoking urges (e.g., distracting attention; changing routines).
Provide basic information – Provide basic information about smoking and successful quitting.	■ The fact that any smoking (even a single puff) increases the likelihood of a full relapse. ■ Withdrawal symptoms typically peak within 1-2 weeks after quitting but may persist for months. These symptoms include negative mood, urges to smoke, and difficulty concentrating. ■ The addictive nature of smoking.

Table 7. Common elements of supportive counseling

Supportive treatment component	Strategies for implementation
Encourage the patient in the quit attempt.	■ Note that effective tobacco dependence treatments are now available. ■ Note that one-half of all people who have ever smoked have now quit. ■ Communicate belief in patient's ability to quit. ■ Encourage patient self-efficacy.
Communicate caring and concern.	■ Ask how patient feels about quitting. ■ Directly express concern and willingness to help as often as needed. ■ Ask about the patient's fears and ambivalence regarding quitting.
Encourage the patient to talk about the quitting process.	Ask about: ■ Reasons the patient wants to quit. ■ Concerns or worries about quitting. ■ Success the patient has achieved. ■ Difficulties encountered while quitting.

Table 8. Providing Counseling—Frequently Asked Questions

My patient doesn't want counseling, only medication. What should I do?	Point out that counseling plus medication works better than medication alone. Explain that the goal of counseling (or coaching) is to provide the practical skills that increase the likelihood of quitting successfully. Use the motivational interventions designed for tobacco users who do not want to quit (see page 24) to encourage your patient to accept counseling. Emphasize the inconsistency between not using effective counseling for something as important and difficult as quitting tobacco. If the patient still declines counseling, consider providing medication alone because medication alone has been shown to be effective. During followup, continue to provide the key elements of counseling: problem solving, practical skills, and support.
My patient wants to use a method of quitting not known to be effective such as acupuncture, hypnosis, or laser therapy. What do I do?	Ask the patient to consider increasing the success odds of his/her quit attempt by augmenting his/her method of quitting with evidence-based medication and counseling. Do not denigrate any attempt to quit. If the patient declines, support his/her effort, but ask for an agreement that, should it not be successful, the patient will consider evidence-based methods in the future, including medication and counseling.
My patient is concerned about gaining weight.	Recommend that the patient start or increase physical activity. For example, take a walk at break time rather than smoke and/or walk at lunch. Also see medication recommendations for such patients.
My patient is concerned about using NRT because he/she believes nicotine to be one of the harmful ingredients in tobacco products.	Explain that medicinal nicotine by itself is relatively safe. Emphasize that the 4,000 chemicals in cigarette smoke, including about 40 carcinogens, cause the harm from smoking. Also, medicinal nicotine has been proven to greatly reduce withdrawal symptoms in many people.

14

Table 8. Providing Counseling—Frequently Asked Questions (continued)

My patient does not want to use medication because of: - **Fear that the medication is addictive** - **Doubt that the medication will help** - **Doubt that recovery is possible if medication containing nicotine is used, having recovered from another dependency.**	Point out: - Medication delivered by mouth or through a patch is not like smoking. Developing a dependency on the medication is uncommon. - The probability of successful quitting is much higher when medication is used. - Substance abuse counselors routinely use medication to help people quit. - The ultimate goal remains neither smoking nor using medication; the use of nicotine-containing medication is a transition step toward that goal. - Consider a medication that does not contain nicotine.
My patient says his/her life is too stressful to quit smoking and he/she needs to smoke to relax.	Acknowledge that for many people smoking is one way to deal with stress. But it is only one way. Counseling will help him/her develop new ways to cope. It will take some time. At first the new ways may feel less effective but the longer the patient is away from smoking, the easier it will be to handle stress without smoking. Also his/her health will be so much better.
My patient says he/she has been smoking for many (20, 30, or more) years without any health problems, plus his/her grandfather smoked two packs a day and lived to be 105.	Consider saying something like, "There are certainly people who smoke for many years without apparent tobacco-related diseases. But about half of people who smoke will die from a tobacco-related illness. The average smoker lives 10 years less than non-smokers. I know it is hard to quit, but is that any reason to gamble with your health when you know that there is a 50-percent chance you will die from a tobacco-related disease?"

Table 9. Suggestions for the clinical use of medication for tobacco dependence treatment[a]

Medication	Cautions/Warnings	Side Effects	Dosage	Use	Availability (check insurance)
Bupropion SR 150	Not for use if you: * Currently use monoamine oxidase (MAO) inhibitor * Use bupropion in any other form * Have a history of seizures * Have a history of eating disorders * See FDA package insert warning regarding suicidality and antidepressant drugs when used in children, adolescents, and young adults.	* Insomnia * Dry mouth	* Days 1-3: 150 mg each morning *Days 4-end: twice daily	Start 1-2 weeks before quit date; use 2 to 6 months	Prescription only * Generic * Zyban * Wellbutrin SR
Nicotine Gum (2 mg or 4 mg)	* Caution with dentures * Do not eat or drink 15 minutes before or during use	* Mouth soreness * Stomach ache	* 1 piece every 1 to 2 hours * 6-15 pieces per day * If ⊡ 24 cigs: 2 mg * If ⊡ 25 cigs/day or chewing tobacco: 4 mg	Up to 12 weeks or as needed	OTC only: * Generic * Nicorette
Nicotine Inhaler	* May irritate mouth/throat at first (but improves with use)	* Local irritation of mouth & throat	* 6-16 cartridges/day * Inhale 80 times/ cartridge * May save partially-used cartridge for next day	Up to 6 months; taper at end	Prescription only: Nicotrol inhaler

16

Table 9. Suggestions for the clinical use of medication for tobacco dependence treatment (continued)[a]

Medication	Cautions/Warnings	Side Effects	Dosage	Use	Availability (check insurance)
Nicotine Lozenge (2 mg or 4 mg)	* Do not eat or drink 15 minutes before or during use * One lozenge at a time * Limit 20 in 24 hours	* Hiccups * Cough * Heartburn	* If smoke/chew 30 minutes after waking: 2 mg * If smoke/chew 30 minutes after waking: 4 mg * Weeks 1-6: 1 every 1-2 hrs * Wks 7-9: 1 every 2-4 hrs * Wks 10-12: 1 every 4-8 hrs	3-6 months	OTC only: * Generic * Commit
Nicotine Nasal Spray	* Not for patients with asthma * May irritate nose (improves over time) * May cause dependence	* Nasal irritation	* 1 "dose" = 1 squirt per nostril 1 to 2 doses per hour * 8 to 40 doses per day * Do NOT inhale	3-6 months; taper at end	Prescription only: * Nicotrol NS

17

Table 9. Suggestions for the clinical use of medication for tobacco dependence treatment (continued)[a]

Medication	Cautions/Warnings	Side Effects	Dosage	Use	Availability (check insurance)
Nicotine Patch	Do not use if you have severe eczema or psoriasis	* Local skin reaction * Insomnia	* One patch per day * If ☒ 10 cigs/day: 21 mg 4 wks, 14 mg 2-4 wks, 7 mg 2-4 wks * If <10/day: 14 mg 4 wks, then 7 mg 4 wks	8-12 weeks	OTC or prescription: * Generic * Nicoderm CQ * Nicotrol
Varenicline	Use with caution in patients: * With significant renal impairment * With serious psychiatric illness * Undergoing dialysis * FDA Warning: Varenicline patients have reported depressed mood, agitation, changes in behavior, suicidal ideation, and suicide. * See www.fda.gov for further updates regarding recommended safe use of Varenicline.	* Nausea * Insomnia * Abnormal, vivid, or strange dreams	* Days 1-3: 0.5 mg every morning * Days 4-7: 0.5 mg twice daily * Day 8-end: 1 mg twice daily	Start 1 week before quit date; use 3-6 months	Prescription only: *Chantix
Combinations: 1) Patch + bupropion 2) Patch + gum 3) Patch + lozenge + inhaler	* Only patch + bupropion is currently FDA approved * Follow instructions for individual medications.	See individual medications above.	See individual medications above.	See above	See above

[a]Based on the 2008 Clinical Practice Guideline: *Treating Tobacco Use and Dependence*, U.S. Public Health Service, May 2008.
See the FDA Web site for additional dosing and safety information, including safety protocols.

18

Table 10. Providing Medication—Frequently Asked Questions

Who should receive medication for tobacco use? Are there groups of smokers for whom medication has not been shown to be effective?	All smokers trying to quit should be offered medication, except where contraindicated or for specific populations for which there is insufficient evidence of effectiveness (i.e., pregnant women, smokeless tobacco users, light smokers, and adolescents).
What are the recommended first-line medications?	All seven of the FDA-approved medications for treating tobacco use are recommended: bupropion SR, nicotine gum, nicotine inhaler, nicotine lozenge, nicotine nasal spray, the nicotine patch, and varenicline. The clinician should consider the first-line medications shown to be more effective than the nicotine patch alone: 2 mg/day varenicline or the combination of long-term nicotine patch use + ad libitum NRT. Unfortunately, there are no well-accepted algorithms to guide optimal selection among the first-line medications.
Are there contraindications, warnings, precautions, other concerns, and side effects regarding the first-line medications recommended in this Guideline Update?	All seven FDA-approved medications have specific contraindications, warnings, precautions, other concerns, and side effects. Please refer to FDA package inserts and updates for complete information on how to use the medication safely.
What other factors may influence medication selection?	Pragmatic factors may also influence selection such as insurance coverage or out-of-pocket patient costs, likelihood of adherence, dentures when considering the gum, or dermatitis when considering the patch.

19

Table 10. Providing Medication—Frequently Asked Questions (continued)

Is a patient's prior experience with a medication relevant?	Prior successful experience (sustained abstinence with the medication) suggests that the medication may be helpful to the patient in a subsequent quit attempt, especially if the patient found the medication to be tolerable and/or easy to use. However, it is difficult to draw firm conclusion from prior failure with a medication. Some evidence suggests that retreating relapsed smokers with the same medication produces small or no benefit while other evidence suggests that it may be of substantial benefit.
What medications should a clinician use with a patient who is highly nicotine dependent?	The higher dose preparations of nicotine gum, patch, and lozenge have been shown to be effective in highly dependent smokers. Also, there is evidence that combination NRT therapy may be particularly effective in suppressing tobacco withdrawal symptoms. Thus, it may be that NRT combinations are especially helpful to highly dependent smokers or those with a history of severe withdrawal.
Is gender a consideration in selecting a medication?	There is evidence that NRT can be effective with both sexes; however, evidence is mixed as to whether NRT is less effective in women than men. This may encourage the clinician to consider use of another type of medication with women such as bupropion SR or varenicline.
Are cessation medications appropriate for light smokers (i.e., <10 cigarettes/ day)?	As noted above, cessation medications have not been shown to be beneficial to light smokers. However, if NRT is used with light smokers, clinicians may consider reducing the dose of the medication. No adjustments are necessary when using bupropion SR or varenicline.

20

Table 10. Providing Medication—Frequently Asked Questions (continued)

When should second-line agents be used for treating tobacco dependence?	Consider prescribing second-line agents (clonidine and nortriptyline) for patients unable to use first-line medications because of contraindications or for patients for whom the group of first-line medications has not been helpful. Assess patients for the specific contraindications, precautions, other concerns, and side effects of the second-line agents. Please refer to FDA package inserts for this information.
Which medications should be considered with patients particularly concerned about weight gain?	Data show that bupropion SR and nicotine replacement therapies, in particular 4 mg nicotine gum and 4 mg nicotine lozenge, delay, but do not prevent, weight gain.
Are there medications that should be especially considered in patients with a past history of depression?	Bupropion SR and nortriptyline appear to be effective with this population, but nicotine replacement medications also appear to help individuals with a past history of depression.
Should nicotine replacement therapies be avoided in patients with a history of cardiovascular disease?	No. The nicotine patch in particular has been demonstrated as safe for cardiovascular patients.
May tobacco dependence medications be used long term (e.g., up to 6 months)?	Yes. This approach may be helpful with smokers who report persistent withdrawal symptoms during the course of medications, who have relapsed in the past after stopping medication, or who desire long-term therapy. A minority of individuals who successfully quit smoking use ad libitum NRT medications (gum, nasal spray, inhaler) long term. The use of these medications for up to 6 months does not present a known health risk and developing dependence on medications is uncommon. Additionally, the FDA has approved the use of bupropion SR, varenicline, and some NRT medications for 6-month use.

21

Table 10. Providing Medication—Frequently Asked Questions (continued)

Is medication adherence important?	Yes. Patients frequently do not use cessation medications as recommended (e.g., they don't use them at recommended doses or for recommended durations); this may reduce their effectiveness.
May medications ever be combined?	Yes. Among first-line medications, evidence exists exists that combining the nicotine patch long term (> 14 weeks) with nicotine gum or nicotine nasal spray, the nicotine patch with the nicotine inhaler, or the nicotine patch with bupropion SR, increases long-term abstinence rates relative to placebo treatments.
My patient can't afford medications and doesn't have insurance to cover it. What can I do?	▪ Instruct the patient to set aside all the money they would have spent on tobacco once they quit. After initial use of medication they will be able to afford medication going forward.
	▪ Many clinics that serve people with no health insurance will provide treatment for tobacco dependence, including medication. Check for ones in your area and have them available for staff and patients as a referral source.
	▪ As a clinician, you can call the tobacco quitline and ask about any sources of free or reduced cost medication for your patients. Try 1-800-QUIT-NOW, which works nationwide and seamlessly routes you to the quitline in the State you are calling from.
	▪ If your patient qualifies for Medicaid or Medicare, these programs cover some tobacco dependence treatment medications. Get this information for your State and have available for staff and patients.
	▪ Most pharmaceutical companies have programs to provide medications to those who cannot afford them. Contact the pharmaceutical companies directly or check with Partnership for Prescription Assistance at www.pparx.org or 1-888-4PPA-NOW.

ARRANGE

Tobacco dependence is an addiction. Quitting is very difficult for most tobacco users. It is essential that the patient trying to quit has scheduled followup. This is especially important when the treatment is shared by a team of clinicians and includes treatment extenders such as quitline counseling.

Table 11. Arrange—Ensure followup contact

Action	Strategies for implementation
Arrange for followup contacts, either in person or via telephone.	*Timing:* Followup contact should begin soon after the quit date, preferably during the first week. A second followup contact is recommended within the first month. Schedule further followup contacts as indicated. *Actions during followup contact:* For all patients, identify problems already encountered and anticipate challenges in the immediate future. Assess medication use and problems. Remind patients of quitline support (1-800-QUIT-NOW). Address tobacco use at next clinical visit (treat tobacco use as a chronic disease). For patients who are abstinent, congratulate them on their success.

23

TOBACCO USERS UNWILLING TO QUIT AT THIS TIME

Ask, Advise, and Assess every tobacco user following the suggestions in Tables 2-4 on pages 8-9. If the patient is unwilling to make a quit attempt at this time, use the motivational strategies that follow to increase the likelihood of quitting in the future.

Assist

Tobacco users who do not want to quit now should be provided with specific interventions designed to increase the likelihood that they will decide to quit. This goal can be achieved through strategies designed to enhance motivation to quit.

Such interventions could incorporate the "5 R's": Relevance, Risk, Rewards, Roadblocks, and Repetition. In these interventions, the clinician can introduce the topic of quitting but it is important that the tobacco users address each topic in their own words. The clinician can then help refine the patient's responses and add to them as needed.

Table 12. Enhancing motivation to quit tobacco—the "5 R's"

Relevance	Encourage the patient to indicate why quitting is personally relevant, being as specific as possible. Motivational information has the greatest impact if it is relevant to a patient's disease status or risk, family or social situation (e.g., having children in the home), health concerns, age, gender, and other important patient characteristics (e.g., prior quitting experience, personal barriers to cessation).
Risks	The clinician should ask the patient to identify potential negative consequences of tobacco use. The clinician may suggest and highlight those that seem most relevant to the patient. The clinician should emphasize that smoking low-tar/low-nicotine cigarettes or use of other forms of tobacco (e.g., smokeless tobacco, cigars, and pipes) will not eliminate these risks. Examples of risks are:
	▪ Acute risks: Shortness of breath, exacerbation of asthma or bronchitis, increased risk of respiratory infections, harm to pregnancy, impotence, infertility.
	▪ Long-term risks: Heart attacks and strokes, lung and other cancers (e.g., larynx, oral cavity, pharynx, esophagus, pancreas, stomach, kidney, bladder, cervix and acute myelocytic leukemia), chronic obstructive pulmonary diseases (chronic bronchitis and emphysema), osteoporosis, long-term disability, and need for extended care.

Table 12. Enhancing motivation to quit tobacco—the "5 R's" (continued)

	▢ Environmental risks: Increased risk of lung cancer and heart disease in spouses; increased risk for low birth weight, sudden infant death syndrome (SIDS), asthma, middle ear disease, and respiratory infections in children of smokers.
Rewards	The clinician should ask the patient to identify potential benefits of stopping tobacco use. The clinician may suggest and highlight those that seem most relevant to the patient. Examples of rewards follow: ▢ Improved health. ▢ Food will taste better. ▢ Improved sense of smell. ▢ Saving money. ▢ Feeling better about yourself. ▢ Home, car, clothing, breath will smell better. ▢ Setting a good example for children and decreasing the likelihood that they will smoke. ▢ Having healthier babies and children. ▢ Feeling better physically. ▢ Performing better in physical activities. ▢ Improved appearance including reduced wrinkling/aging of skin and whiter teeth.
Roadblocks	The clinician should ask the patient to identify barriers or impediments to quitting and provide treatment (problem-solving counseling, medication) that could address barriers. Typical barriers might include: ▢ Withdrawal symptoms. ▢ Fear of failure. ▢ Weight gain. ▢ Lack of support. ▢ Depression. ▢ Enjoyment of tobacco. ▢ Being around other tobacco users. ▢ Limited knowledge of effective treatment options.
Repetition	The motivational intervention should be repeated every time an unmotivated patient visits the clinic setting. Tobacco users who have failed in previous quit attempts should be told that most people make repeated quit attempts before they are successful and that you will continue to raise their tobacco use with them.

Interventions to increase the likelihood that a tobacco user who does not want to quit will decide to quit can draw upon the principles of motivational interviewing:

Table 13. Motivational interviewing strategies

Express Empathy	▪ Use open-ended questions to explore:
	o The importance of addressing smoking or other tobacco use (e.g., "How important do you think it is for you to quit?").
	o Concerns and benefits of quitting (e.g., "What might happen if you quit?").
	▪ Use reflective listening to seek shared understanding:
	o Reflect words or meaning (e.g., "So you think smoking helps you to maintain your weight?").
	o Summarize (e.g., "What I have heard so far is that smoking is something you enjoy. On the other hand, your boyfriend hates your smoking and you are worried you might develop a serious disease.").
	▪ Normalize feelings and concerns (e.g., "Many people worry about managing without cigarettes.")
	▪ Support the patient's autonomy and right to choose or reject change (e.g., "I hear you saying you are not ready to quit smoking right now. I'm here to help you when you are ready.")
Develop Discrepancy	▪ Highlight the discrepancy between the patient's present behavior and expressed priorities, values, and goals (e.g., "It sounds like you are very devoted to your family. How do you think your smoking is affecting your children and spouse/partner?").
	▪ Reinforce and support "change talk" and "commitment" language.
	o "So, you realize how smoking is affecting your breathing and making it hard to keep up with your kids."
	o "It's great that you are going to quit when you get through this busy time at work."
	▪ Build and deepen commitment to change
	o "There are effective treatments that will ease the pain of quitting, including counseling and many medication options."
	o "We would like to help you avoid a stroke like the one your father had."

Table 13. Motivational Interviewing Strategies (continued)

Roll with Resistance	▪ Back off and use reflection when the patient expresses resistance.
	o "Sounds like you are feeling pressured about your tobacco use."
	▪ Express empathy.
	o "You are worried about how you would manage withdrawal symptoms."
	▪ Ask permission to provide information.
	o "Would you like to hear about some strategies that can help you address that concern when you quit?"
Support Self-Efficacy	▪ Help the patient to identify and build on past successes.
	o "So you were fairly successful the last time you tried to quit."
	▪ Offer options for achievable, small steps toward change.
	o Call the quitline (1-800-QUIT-NOW) for advice and information.
	o Read about quitting benefits and strategies.
	o Change smoking patterns (e.g., no smoking in the home).
	o Ask the patient to share his or her ideas about quitting strategies.

ARRANGE FOLLOWUP

More than one motivational intervention may be required before the tobacco user who is unwilling to quit commits to a quit attempt. It is essential that the patient trying to quit has scheduled followup. Provide followup at the next visit and additional interventions to motivate and support the decisionmaking process of the patient who is unwilling to quit now.

TOBACCO USERS WHO RECENTLY QUIT

Ask every patient at every visit if they use tobacco and his or her status document-ed clearly in the clinical record (e.g., as part of the vital signs, displayed prominently in the electronic medical record). (See Table 2 for more details)

Table 14. Assess former tobacco user relapse potential

Action	Strategies for implementation
How long has it been since you quit?	Most relapse occurs within the first 2 weeks after the quit date and the risk decreases over time. Tobacco users who have quit very recently should be provided assistance. But the risk for relapse can persist for a long time for many tobacco users. Therefore, assess all former tobacco users, regardless of how long ago they quit, about challenges by asking the question below:
Do you still have any urges to use tobacco or any challenges to remaining tobacco free?	Any recent quitter or former tobacco users still experiencing challenges should receive assistance.

Table 15. Assist former tobacco users with encouragement to stay abstinent

Action	Strategies for implementation
The former tobacco user should receive congratulations on any success and strong encouragement to remain abstinent.	When encountering a recent quitter, use open-ended questions relevant to the topics below to discover if the patient wishes to discuss issues related to quitting: • The benefits, including potential health benefits, the patient may derive from cessation. • Any success the patient has had in quitting (duration of abstinence, reduction in withdrawal, and so on). • The problems encountered or anticipated threats to maintaining abstinence (e.g., depression, weight gain, alcohol, other tobacco users in the household, significant stressors). • A medication check-in, including effectiveness and adherence

Table 16. Specific challenges and potential responses to the tobacco user who recently quit

Challenges	Responses
Lack of support for cessation	• Schedule followup visits or telephone calls with the patient. • Urge the patient to call the quitline (1-800-QUIT-NOW). • Help the patient identify sources of support within his or her environment.
Negative mood or depression	• Refer the patient to an appropriate organization that offers counseling or evidence-based support. • If significant, provide counseling, prescribe appropriate medication, or refer the patient to a specialist.
Strong or prolonged withdrawal symptoms	• If the patient reports prolonged craving or other withdrawal symptoms, consider extending the use of an approved medication or adding/combining medications to reduce strong withdrawal symptoms.
Weight gain	• Recommend starting or increasing physical activity. • Reassure the patient that some weight gain after quitting is common and is usually self-limiting. • Emphasize the health benefits of quitting relative to the health risks of modest weight gain. • Emphasize the importance of a healthy diet and active lifestyle. • Suggest low-calorie substitutes such as sugarless chewing gum, vegetables, or mints. • Maintain the patient on medication known to delay weight gain (e.g., bupropion SR, NRTs, particularly 4 mg nicotine gum, and lozenge). • Refer the patient to a nutritional counselor or program.
Smoking lapses	• Suggest continued use of medications, which can reduce the likelihood that a lapse will lead to a full relapse. • Encourage another quit attempt or a recommitment to total abstinence. • Reassure that quitting may take multiple attempts, and use the lapse as a learning experience • Provide or refer for intensive counseling.

ARRANGE FOLLOWUP

All patients that have recently quit or still face challenges should receive followup for continued assistance and support.

New Recommendations in the PHS–Sponsored Clinical Practice Guideline—*Treating Tobacco Use and Dependence: 2008 Update*

Most, but not all, of the new recommendations appearing in the 2008 Update of the Guideline resulted from new meta-analyses of the topics chosen by the Guideline panel.

1. Formats of Psychosocial Treatments

Recommendation: Tailored materials, both print and Web-based, appear to be effective in helping people quit. Therefore, clinicians may choose to provide tailored, self-help materials to their patients who want to quit.

2. Combining Counseling and Medication

Recommendation: The combination of counseling and medication is more effective for smoking cessation than either medication or counseling alone. Therefore, whenever feasible and appropriate, both counseling and medication should be provided to patients trying to quit smoking.

Recommendation: There is a strong relation between the number of sessions of counseling when it is combined with medication and the likelihood of successful smoking abstinence. Therefore, to the extent possible, clinicians should provide multiple counseling sessions, in addition to medication, to their patients who are trying to quit smoking.

3. For Tobacco Users Not Willing To Quit Now

Recommendation: Motivational intervention techniques appear to be effective in increasing a patient's likelihood of making a future quit attempt. Therefore, clinicians should use motivational techniques to encourage smokers who are not currently willing to quit to consider making a quit attempt in the future.

4. Nicotine Lozenge

Recommendation: The nicotine lozenge is an effective smoking cessation treatment that patients should be encouraged to use.
Note: See the Guideline and FDA Web site (www.fda.gov) for additional information on the safe and effective use of medication.

5. Varenicline

Recommendation: Varenicline is an effective smoking cessation treatment that patients should be encouraged to use.
Note: See the Guideline and the FDA Web site (www.fda.gov) for additional information on the safe and effective use of medication.

6. Specific Populations

Recommendation: The interventions found to be effective in this Guideline have been shown to be effective in a variety of populations. In addition, many of the studies supporting these interventions comprised diverse samples of tobacco users. Therefore, interventions identified as effective in this Guideline are recommended for all individuals who use tobacco except when medically contraindicated or with specific populations in which medication has not been shown to be effective (pregnant women, smokeless tobacco users, light (< 10 cigarettes/day) smokers, and adolescents).

7. Light Smokers

Recommendation: Light smokers should be identified, strongly urged to quit and provided counseling treatment interventions.

Conclusion

Tobacco dependence is a chronic disease that deserves treatment. Effective treatments have now been identified and should be used with every current and former smoker. This Quick Reference Guide for Clinicians provides clinicians with the tools necessary to effectively identify and assess tobacco use and to treat (1) tobacco users willing to quit, (2) those who are unwilling to quit at this time, and (3) former tobacco users. There is no clinical treatment available today that can reduce illness, prevent death, and increase quality of life more than effective tobacco treatment interventions.

Guideline Availability

The Guideline is available in several formats suitable for health care practitioners, the scientific community, educators, and consumers.

The Clinical Practice Guideline—*Treating Tobacco Use and Dependence: 2008 Update* presents recommendations for health care providers with supporting information, tables, and figures.

The *Quick Reference Guide for Clinicians* is a distilled version of the clinical practice guideline, with summary points for ready reference daily.

Helping Smokers Quit: A Guide for Clinicians is a pocket guide that presents a brief summary of the 5 A's, including a chart regarding medications.

Help for Smokers and Other Tobacco Users is an informational booklet designed for tobacco users with limited formal education.

The full text of the guideline documents, references, and the meta-analyses references for online retrieval are available by visiting the Surgeon General's Web Site: www.surgeongeneral.gov/tobacco/default.htm

Single copies of these guideline products and further information on the availability of other derivative products can be obtained by calling any of the following Public Health Service clearinghouses toll-free numbers:

Agency for Healthcare Research and Quality (AHRQ)
800-358-9295

Centers for Disease Control and Prevention (CDC)
800-CDC-1311

National Cancer Institute (NCI)
800-4-CANCER

CPSIA information can be obtained
at www.ICGtesting.com
Printed in the USA
BVOW06s2111160317
478711BV00014B/92/P

9 781490 500461